5 Minute Yoga: Quick Daily Practices for Busy Lives

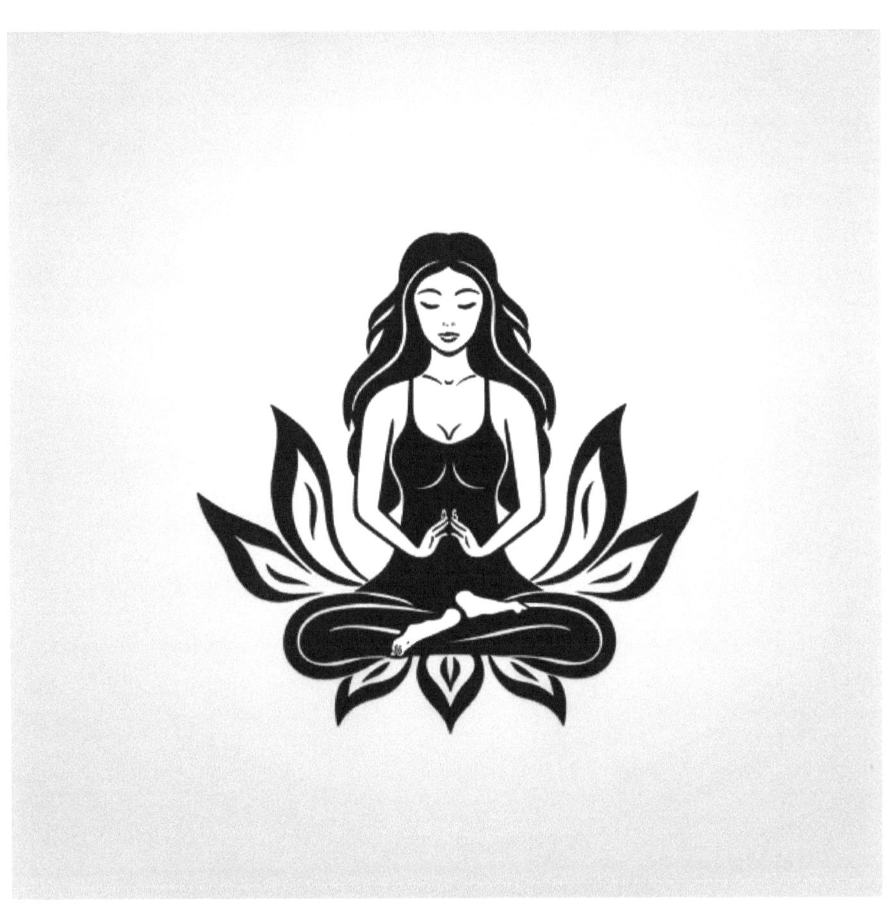

Janet Nagajew

Introduction

Hello there! Welcome to "5 Minute Yoga: Quick Daily Practices for Busy Lives." I've created this book to demystify yoga and make it accessible for everyone, no matter how jam-packed your schedule might be.

Yoga, an ancient practice that intertwines the mind, body, and spirit, is just as useful in our modern world as it was thousands of years ago. Yet, with the hectic pace of life today, finding the time to engage in a long yoga session can be daunting. That's where this guide comes in, offering yoga that fits your busy life.

In the pages that follow, we'll cut to the chase, offering you the key elements of yoga in digestible, manageable pieces. I'll introduce you to the core principles of yoga, present you with eight distinct, short, but effective yoga sequences, and guide you on customizing these practices for specific needs, whether it's stress relief, better sleep, energy boost, or improved posture. Plus, I'll share my personal tips on building a consistent yoga routine, regardless of how hectic your day might be.

This book isn't aimed at turning you into a yoga guru. Instead, it's a practical, friendly guide to help you make yoga a part of your everyday life. Just by dedicating five minutes a day, you'll notice a world of difference in your physical health, mental clarity, and overall sense of well-being.

So, whether you're an absolute beginner, a busy professional, a parent, or anyone looking for a healthier life, this book is for you. It's time to unroll that yoga mat, carve out five minutes from your day, and begin this rewarding journey. Let's dive in!

Understanding Yoga

Yoga, with its roots stretching back over 5,000 years, is an ancient practice that originated in the Indian subcontinent. The term 'yoga' is derived from the Sanskrit word 'yuj', which means to unite or bind, often interpreted as "union". Initially, yoga was a spiritual path, a way to achieve harmony between the heart and soul, leading to divine enlightenment. As time passed, yoga has evolved and adapted, taking on various forms and interpretations across different cultures and societies.

The ancient yogic seers, known as 'rishis', perceived the mind and body as one interconnected whole. They proposed that to attain a state of inner peace and self-realization, one must harmonize the physical, mental, and spiritual aspects of existence. This comprehensive approach forms the bedrock of yoga and is mirrored in its fundamental principles.

Yoga is grounded in six key principles: proper relaxation, proper exercise (asanas), proper breathing (pranayama), proper diet, positive thinking and meditation, and proper rest. Asanas, or poses, are designed to enhance body flexibility and strength. Pranayama, or controlled breathing, is used to soothe the mind, improve focus, and manage stress. Meditation, the practice of concentrating the mind to achieve tranquility, is a cornerstone of yoga, promoting mental clarity and self-awareness.

Over the centuries, yoga has undergone significant evolution. It has transitioned from a spiritual practice aimed at enlightenment to a comprehensive health practice focusing on mental and physical well-being. Today, there are various styles of yoga, each with its unique focus and methodology, ranging from the physically intense Ashtanga and Vinyasa styles to the more meditative and restorative styles like Yin and Restorative yoga.

Yoga offers a plethora of physical and mental benefits, many of which are well-documented. Physically, yoga can enhance flexibility, muscle strength, and body tone. It can boost respiration, energy, and vitality. Regular yoga practice can also help maintain a balanced metabolism, promote cardiovascular and circulatory health, improve athletic performance, and offer protection from injury.

Mentally, yoga is a powerful tool for managing stress, which can wreak havoc on the body and mind. Stress can manifest in many ways, including back or neck pain, sleeping problems, headaches, drug abuse, and an inability to concentrate. Yoga can be highly effective in developing coping skills and fostering a more positive outlook on life. Yoga's combination of meditation and breathing can significantly improve a person's mental well-being. Regular yoga practice fosters mental clarity and calmness, increases body awareness, alleviates chronic stress patterns, relaxes the mind, centers attention, and sharpens concentration.

Numerous studies have corroborated these benefits. For instance, a study published in the Journal of Physical Activity and Health found that 20 minutes of Hatha yoga stimulates brain function more than walking or jogging on the treadmill for the same duration. Another study published in the Journal of Alternative and Complementary Medicine discovered that yoga helps improve balance and mobility in older adults. Yet another study found that practicing yoga could help reduce inflammation, the body's response to injury or irritation, which is linked to a host of health issues including heart disease, diabetes, and cancer.

In conclusion, yoga is a comprehensive practice that promotes physical health, mental clarity, and spiritual growth. Its principles and practices have withstood the test of time and continue to be relevant in our modern world. Whether you're seeking physical fitness, stress relief, or spiritual enlightenment, yoga has something to offer.

Disclaimer

This book is here to provide you with useful and insightful information about yoga. However, it's not a substitute for professional medical advice or treatment. If you have a medical condition, or if you're not sure about your health status, please consult with your doctor before starting any new exercise program, including the yoga practices outlined in this book.

The author and publisher of this book can't be held responsible for any health issues or allergies that might require medical attention. We're also not liable for any harm or negative outcomes from any treatment, action, or preparation that a reader might decide to take based on the information provided in this book.

It's really important to be in good health before you start any exercise program, and yoga is no different. So, before you start practicing the yoga sequences in this book, please get a green light from a healthcare professional.

The yoga exercises described in this book should be attempted at your own risk. If something doesn't feel right, or if you experience any discomfort or pain, stop immediately. The advice and instructions given in this book are not meant to replace medical or psychological counseling.

Remember, safety first. Always practice in a calm and peaceful environment, and listen to your body. It's your best guide.

Getting Started

As you step onto the yoga mat for the first time, there are a few basic terms you'll come across quite often. These words, rooted in the ancient language of Sanskrit, are part of the common language in yoga classes and literature.

"Asana": Simply put, asana means pose or posture. When you hear the term asana, it refers to the physical poses you'll be practicing in yoga. For instance, "Tadasana" is what we call the Mountain Pose, which is great for improving your posture, and "Savasana" is the Corpse Pose, a relaxing posture usually done at the end of a yoga session.

"Pranayama": This term is a combination of 'Prana', which means life force or breath, and 'ayama', meaning control or extension. So, pranayama is all about controlling and extending your breath. It's a set of breathing exercises that help control the energy within your body using your breath.

"Vinyasa": Vinyasa is a style of yoga where you move from one pose to another smoothly, coordinating your movements with your breath. It's almost like a dance, where each movement is tied to an inhale or exhale.

Now that we've covered some basic terms, let's talk about the importance of posture, alignment, and safety.

Posture and alignment are key in yoga. They ensure that you're doing each pose correctly, getting the most out of it, and not risking injury. Here are some basic tips:

Keep your body aligned. In standing poses, your hips should be lined up with your ankles. In seated poses, your hips should be aligned with your knees.

Don't push yourself too hard. Yoga isn't about touching your toes or doing the most difficult poses. It's about connecting your mind, body, and breath. Always listen to your body and respect its limits.

Don't be afraid to use props. Things like yoga blocks, straps, and bolsters can help you achieve the correct alignment and make poses more comfortable.

Always warm up before starting your practice. Like any other physical activity, it's important to warm up your body before starting yoga. This could be a few simple stretches or a couple of rounds of Sun Salutations.

Finish your practice with Savasana or Corpse Pose. This pose allows your body and mind to absorb the benefits of your practice.

Breathing is a vital part of yoga. It connects the mind and body, helps you stay focused, and drives your movements and transitions between poses. Here's a simple breathing exercise for beginners, known as "Three-Part Breath" or "Dirga Pranayama":

Find a comfortable seated position. Close your eyes and start to notice your natural breath.

Place one hand on your belly and the other on your chest. As you inhale, fill your belly with air, then let the breath rise to expand your rib cage and finally, fill your chest. As you exhale, let the breath go first from the chest, then the rib cage, and finally, let the belly draw in towards the spine.

Continue this pattern for a few minutes, taking slow and deep breaths, fully filling and emptying your lungs.

Remember, yoga is a personal journey. It's not about perfection but progress. Listen to your body, respect its limits, and most importantly, enjoy the practice.

Sequence One: Building Core Strength

Introduction and Overview

Having a strong core is like having a sturdy anchor for your body. It's not just about getting toned abs; it's about enhancing your balance, supporting your spine, and making daily activities easier. This sequence is designed to help you build that strong core, boosting your overall fitness and well-being.

Boat Pose (Navasana)

The Boat Pose is like a mini workout for your abs and hip flexors. It's a fantastic pose to kickstart our core-strengthening journey.

Instructions:

Sit on your mat, bend your knees and keep your feet flat on the floor.
Lean back slightly, lift your feet off the floor, and balance on your sit bones.
Extend your arms in front of you, keeping them parallel to the floor.
If you can, straighten your legs so that your toes are at eye level.
Modifications: If you find it hard to straighten your legs, no worries! Keep your knees bent.
You can also place your hands on the floor behind you for extra support.

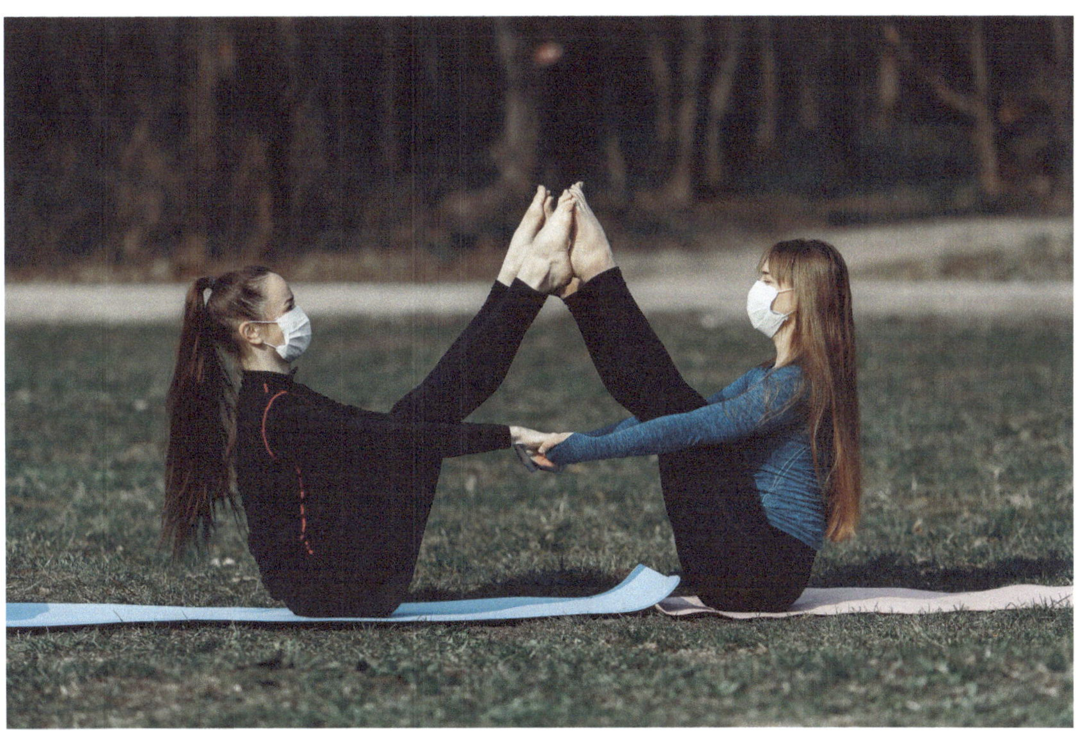

Plank Pose (Kumbhakasana)
The Plank Pose is like the superhero of yoga poses. It works your entire body, with a special emphasis on the core.

Instructions:

Start on all fours, making sure your wrists are directly under your shoulders.
Extend your legs behind you, coming onto the balls of your feet.
Engage your core and make sure your body forms a straight line from your head to your heels.
Modifications: If holding a full plank feels too tough, lower your knees to the floor. You're still a superhero!

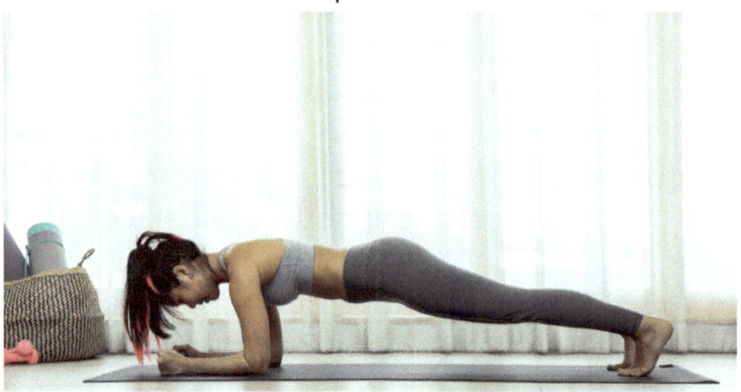

Bridge Pose (Setu Bandha Sarvangasana)
The Bridge Pose is a great way to strengthen your back and abdominal muscles, while also opening up your chest and shoulders.

Instructions:

Lie on your back with your knees bent and feet flat on the floor. Keep your arms by your sides.
Press your feet and arms into the floor and lift your hips towards the ceiling.
Make sure your thighs stay parallel to each other and your knees are directly over your ankles.
Modifications: If lifting your hips feels a bit tricky, use a yoga block or bolster under your sacrum for support.

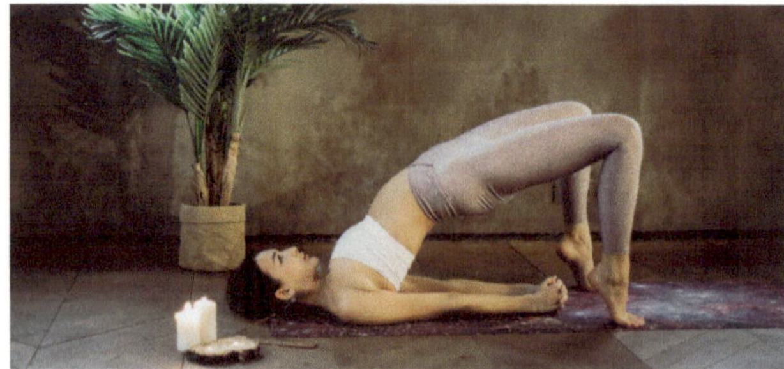

Remember, yoga isn't about perfecting the pose; it's about how you feel while doing it. Always listen to your body and adjust the poses as needed. With regular practice, you'll notice your core getting stronger and your overall fitness improving. Enjoy the Journey.

Sequence Two: Improving Flexibility

Introduction and Overview

Flexibility is more than just being able to touch your toes. It's about having a full range of motion in your joints and muscles, which can help prevent injuries, improve your posture, and even reduce muscle soreness. This sequence is designed to help you gently stretch and lengthen your muscles, enhancing your overall flexibility.

Forward Bend (Uttanasana)
The Forward Bend is a simple yet effective pose that stretches your hamstrings and back muscles.

Instructions:

Stand tall with your feet hip-width apart.
As you exhale, hinge at your hips and fold forward, reaching your hands towards the floor.
Keep your knees slightly bent if you need to.
Modifications: If you can't touch the floor, don't worry! Just let your hands hang down or rest them on your shins.

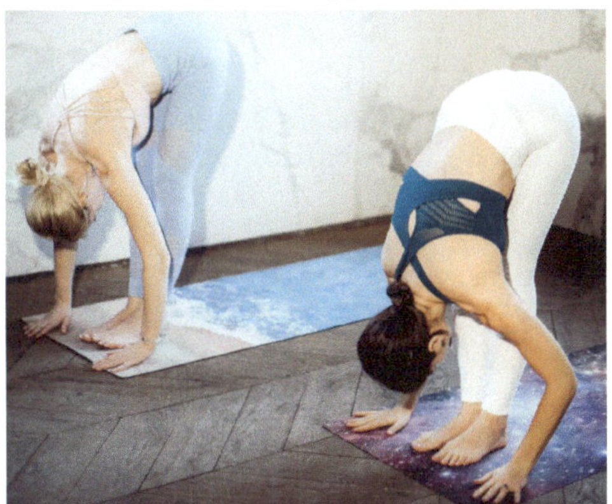

Seated Forward Bend (Paschimottanasana)
The Seated Forward Bend is a great pose for stretching your spine and the back of your body.

Instructions:

Sit on your mat with your legs extended in front of you.
Inhale and reach your arms up towards the ceiling.
As you exhale, hinge at your hips and fold forward, reaching your hands towards your feet.
Modifications: If you can't reach your feet, hold onto your shins or ankles instead.

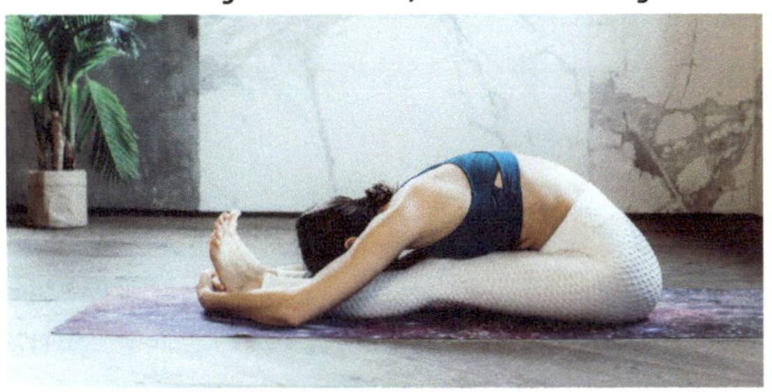

Cobra Pose (Bhujangasana)
The Cobra Pose is a gentle backbend that stretches your chest and abdominal muscles.

Instructions:

Lie on your stomach with your hands under your shoulders.
Press your hands into the mat and lift your chest off the floor, keeping your hips and legs grounded.
Keep a slight bend in your elbows and open your chest forward.
Modifications: If this feels too intense, you can keep your forearms on the ground for a gentler backbend.

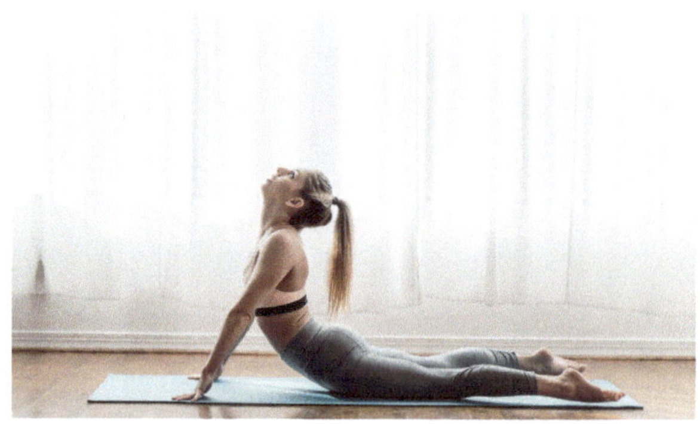

Child's Pose (Balasana)
The Child's Pose is a restful pose that stretches your back, hips, and thighs.

Instructions:

Kneel on your mat with your knees wider than hip-width apart.
Sit back on your heels and fold forward, extending your arms in front of you and resting your forehead on the mat.
Modifications: If your forehead doesn't reach the mat, you can stack your fists or use a block to support it.

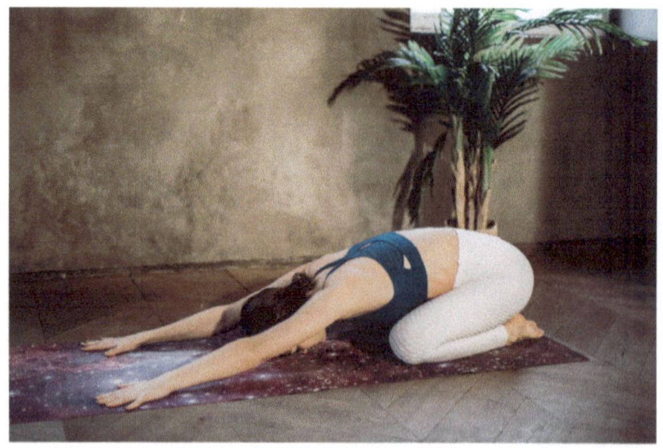

Remember, flexibility doesn't come overnight, but with regular practice, you'll see progress.
Always listen to your body and only stretch as far as feels comfortable. Enjoy the journey

Sequence Three: Promoting Relaxation and Stress Relief

Introduction and Overview

In our fast-paced world, stress can often feel like a constant companion. But did you know that yoga can be a powerful tool for stress relief? This sequence is designed to help you unwind, relax, and let go of stress, bringing a sense of calm and tranquility to your mind and body.

Child's Pose (Balasana)

The Child's Pose is a restful pose that allows you to turn inward and focus on your breath, helping to calm your mind.

Instructions:

Start by kneeling on your mat, with your knees wider than your hips.
Sit back on your heels and fold forward, extending your arms in front of you.
Rest your forehead on the mat and breathe deeply.
Modifications: If your forehead doesn't reach the mat, you can stack your fists or use a block to support it.

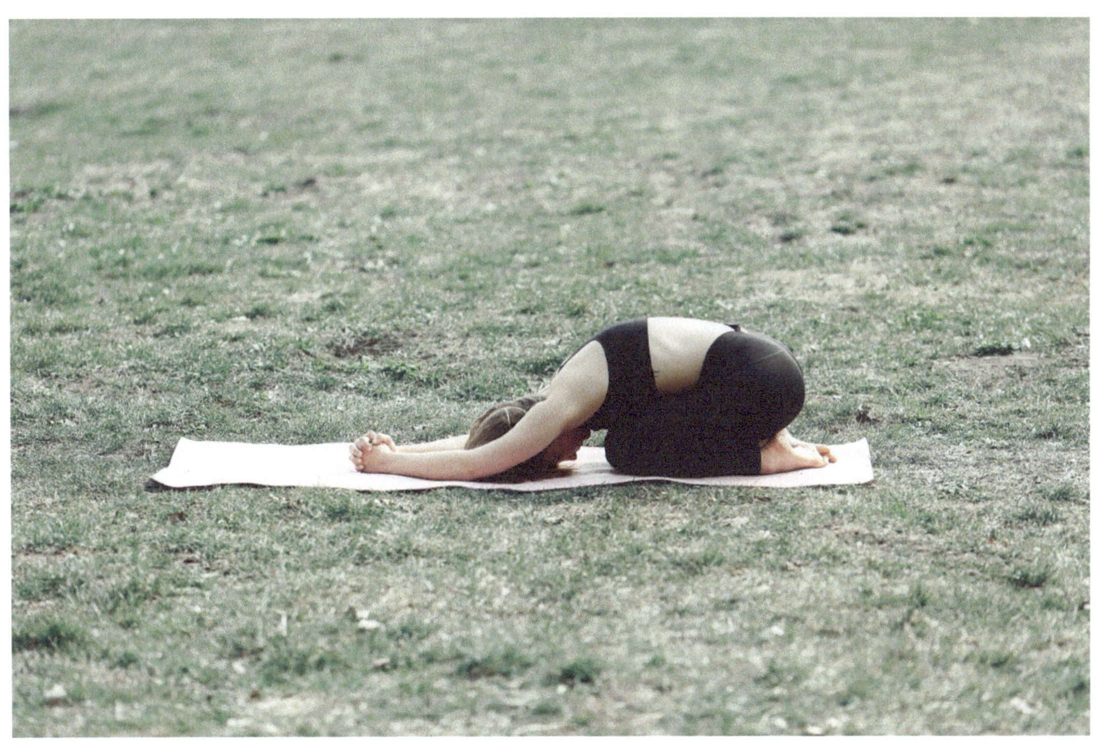

Legs-Up-The-Wall Pose (Viparita Karani)
The Legs-Up-The-Wall Pose is a gentle inversion that helps to relax the body and mind,
making it perfect for stress relief.

Instructions:

Sit sideways against a wall.
Swing your legs up onto the wall as you lean back and lie down on your mat.
Extend your arms out to the sides and relax into the pose.
Modifications: If your hamstrings are tight, you can move a little further away from the wall or
bend your knees slightly.

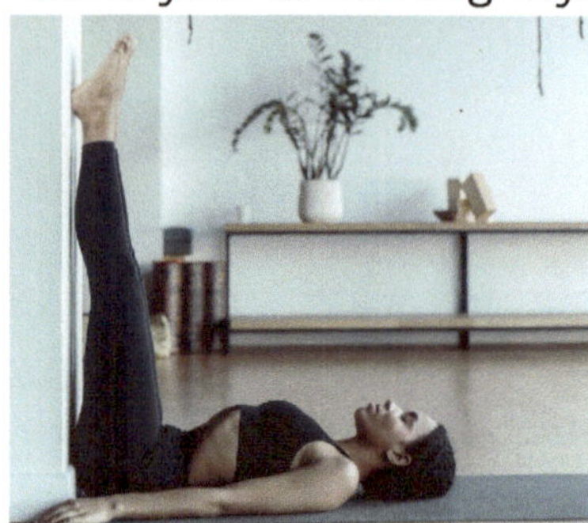

Corpse Pose (Savasana)
The Corpse Pose is typically the final pose in a yoga practice, allowing your body and mind to
absorb the benefits of your practice.

Instructions:

Lie down on your back and let your legs and arms relax, with your palms facing up.
Close your eyes and take slow, deep breaths, allowing your body to relax and sink into the
mat.
Modifications: If lying flat on your back is uncomfortable, you can place a rolled-up blanket or
bolster under your knees.

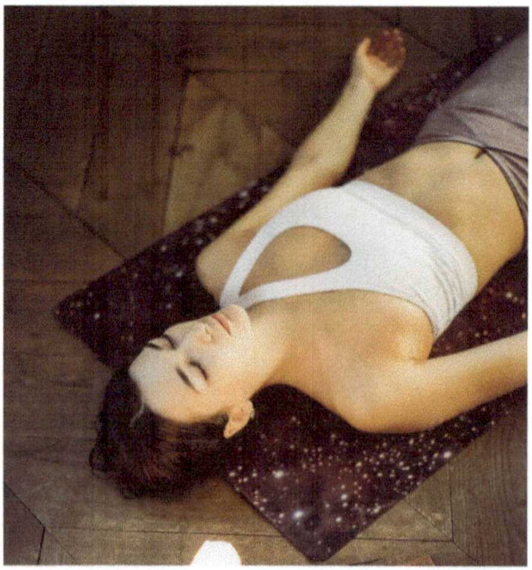

Remember, the goal of this sequence is relaxation and stress relief, so take your time and
move at your own pace. Allow your breath to guide you and let go of any tension with each
exhale. Enjoy the sense of calm and tranquility that comes with your practice.

Sequence Four: Enhancing Balance and Stability

Introduction and Overview

Balance isn't just about standing on one foot without falling over. It's about stability and control, which are crucial for everything from walking and running to bending over and lifting objects. This sequence is designed to help you improve your balance and stability, enhancing your coordination and reducing the risk of falls.

Tree Pose (Vrksasana)

The Tree Pose is a classic balance pose that also strengthens your legs and core.

Instructions:

Stand tall with your feet hip-width apart.
Shift your weight onto your right foot and bring the sole of your left foot to your inner right thigh or calf.
Bring your hands together at your heart or reach them up towards the sky.
Focus on a point in front of you and breathe deeply.
Modifications: If balancing on one foot is challenging, you can keep your toes on the floor with your heel resting on your ankle.

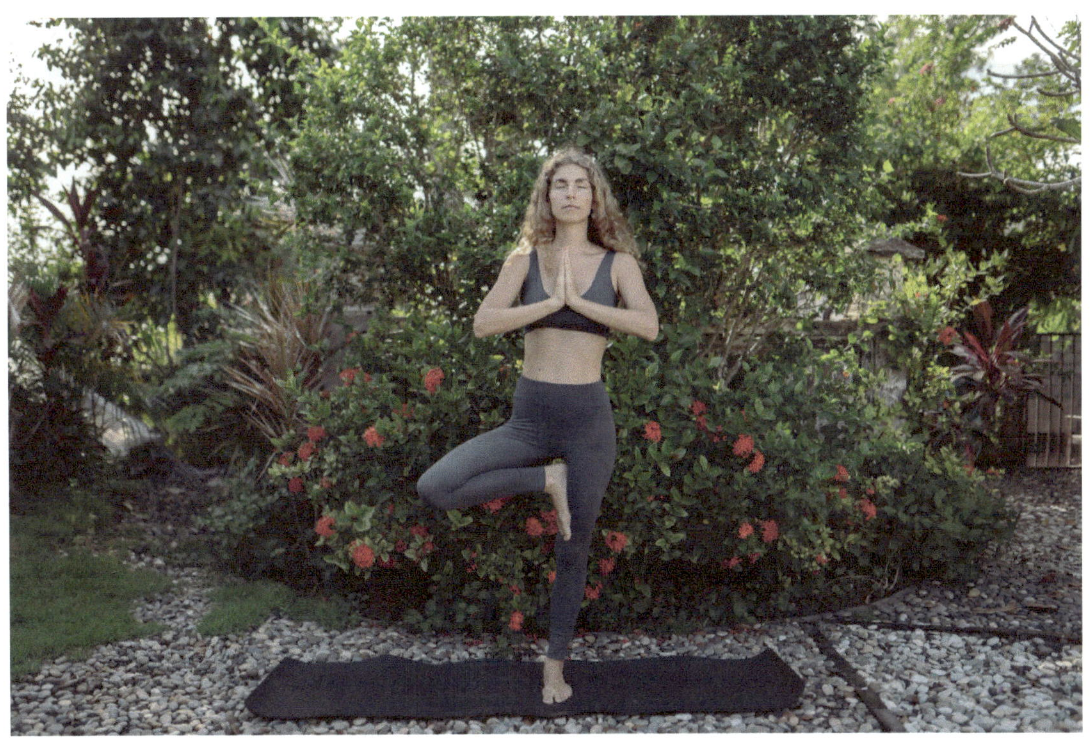

Warrior III (Virabhadrasana III)
The Warrior III pose challenges your balance while strengthening your entire body.

Instructions:

From a standing position, extend your right leg behind you as you lean your torso forward, coming into a "T" shape.
Extend your arms in front of you or alongside your body.
Engage your core and keep your gaze down for balance.
Modifications: You can use a chair or wall for support, or keep your back toes on the ground.

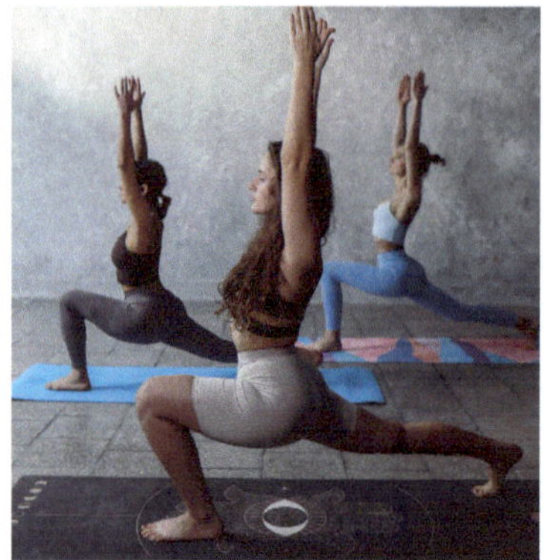

Half Moon Pose (Ardha Chandrasana)
The Half Moon Pose is a dynamic balance pose that also stretches your hamstrings and strengthens your ankles.

Instructions:

From a standing position, lean forward and place your right hand on the ground or a block.
Lift your left leg off the ground and open your hips and chest to the left, reaching your left arm up.
Look up towards your left hand if it feels comfortable for your neck.
Modifications: You can use a block under your hand or keep your gaze down for better balance.

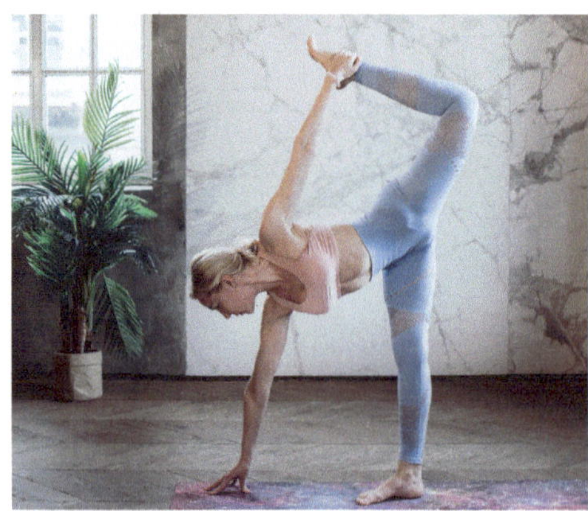

Remember, balance is a skill that improves with practice. Don't worry if you wobble or fall - it's all part of the journey. Just keep trying, and you'll see progress over time. Enjoy the process!

Sequence Five: Boosting Energy Levels

Introduction and Overview

Ever feel like you're running on empty? We all have those days. But the good news is, yoga can help. Certain poses can stimulate your body and mind, giving you a much-needed energy boost. This sequence is designed to help you shake off fatigue and put a spring back in your step.

Sun Salutations (Surya Namaskar)

Sun Salutations are a series of poses that warm up the body and get the energy flowing.

Instructions:

Stand tall at the top of your mat. As you inhale, reach your arms up towards the sky.
As you exhale, fold forward over your legs.
Inhale to a flat back, then exhale and step or jump back to a plank pose.
Lower down to your belly, then inhale to a cobra pose.
Exhale to downward facing dog, then step or jump your feet to your hands.
Inhale to a flat back, then exhale and fold forward.
Inhale and reach your arms up to the sky, then exhale and bring your hands to your heart.
Modifications: Feel free to bend your knees in the forward fold, or keep your knees on the ground in the plank pose.

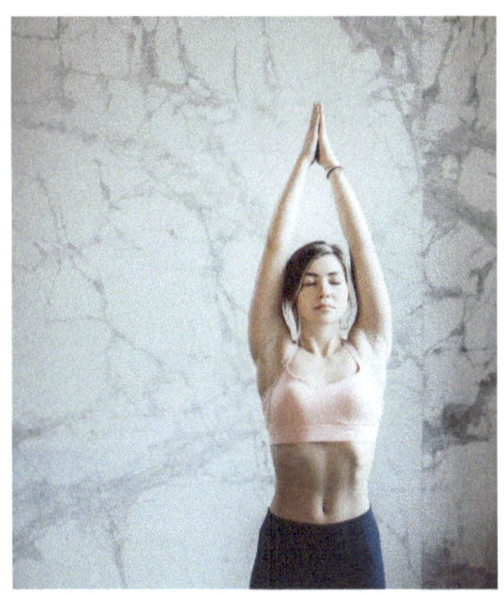
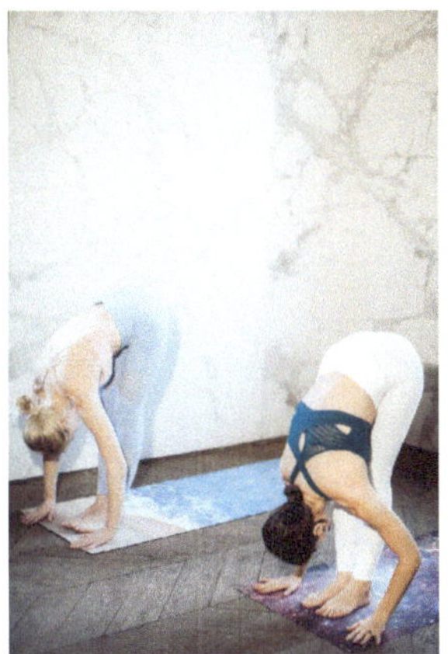
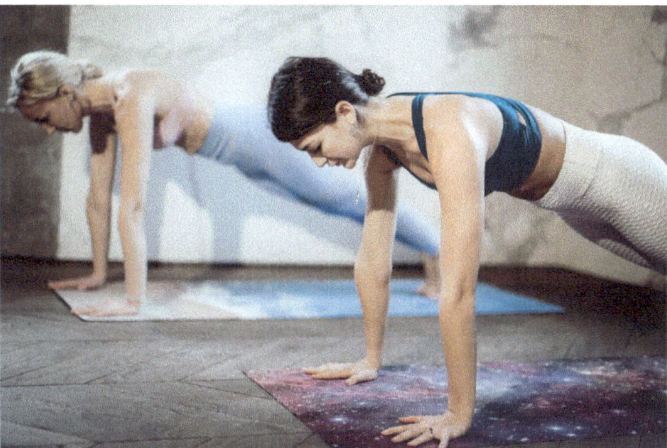
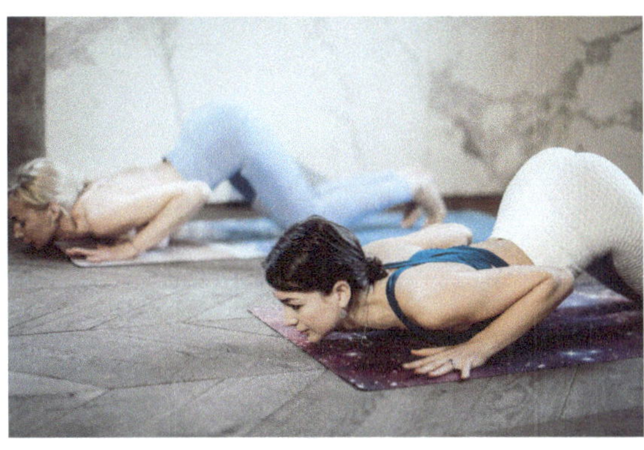
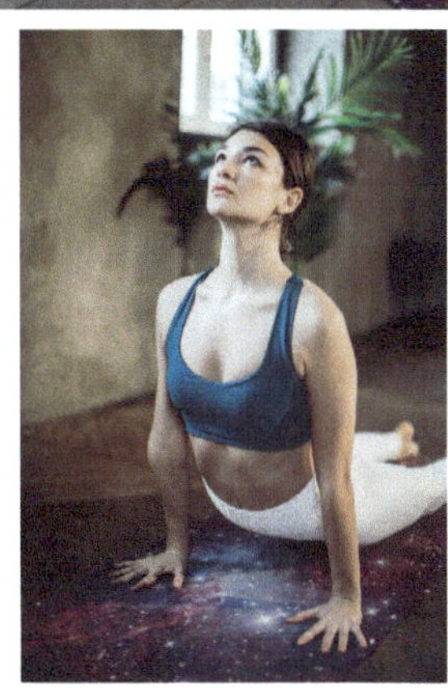

Warrior II (Virabhadrasana II)

Warrior II is a powerful pose that strengthens your legs and ignites your inner warrior.

Instructions:

Stand with your feet wide apart on your mat.
Turn your right foot out and your left foot in slightly.
Bend your right knee and extend your arms out to the sides, gazing over your right hand.
Engage your core and feel the energy radiating out from your center.
Modifications: If your legs get tired, you can straighten your front knee a little.

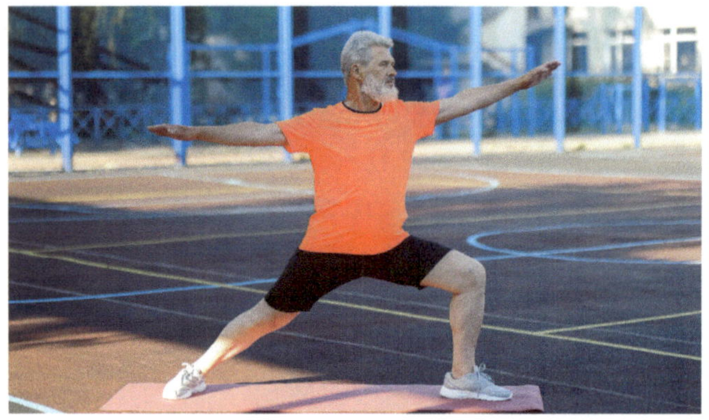

Camel Pose (Ustrasana)

The Camel Pose is a backbend that opens up your chest and boosts your energy.

Instructions:

Kneel on your mat with your knees hip-width apart.
Place your hands on your lower back, fingers pointing down.
Lift your chest up towards the sky as you lean back, keeping your hips over your knees.
If it feels comfortable, you can reach your hands back to your heels.
Modifications: If reaching for your heels is too much, you can keep your hands on your lower back.

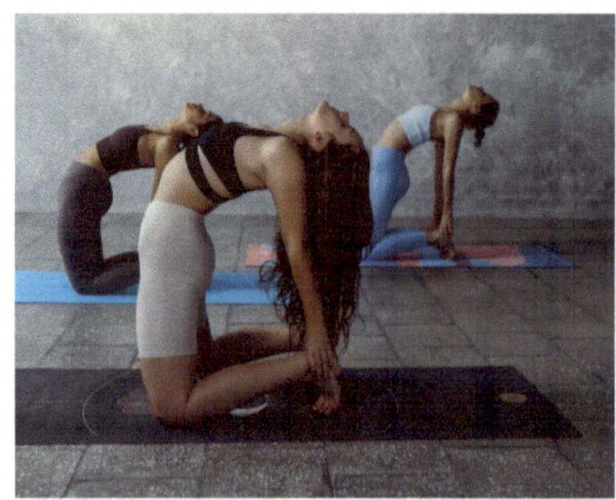

Remember, yoga is all about listening to your body. If you ever feel tired or dizzy, take a break and rest in Child's Pose. And most importantly, enjoy the energy boost and the positive vibes that come with your practice!

Sequence Six: Promoting Better Sleep

Introduction and Overview

Having trouble sleeping? You're not alone. Many of us struggle to get a good night's sleep. But the good news is, yoga can help. This sequence is designed to calm your mind and relax your body, preparing you for a restful night's sleep.

Legs-Up-The-Wall Pose (Viparita Karani)
The Legs-Up-The-Wall Pose is a restorative pose that helps to relax the body and mind.

Instructions:

Sit sideways against a wall.
Swing your legs up onto the wall as you lean back and lie down on your mat.
Extend your arms out to the sides and relax into the pose.
Modifications: If your hamstrings are tight, you can move a little further away from the wall or bend your knees slightly.

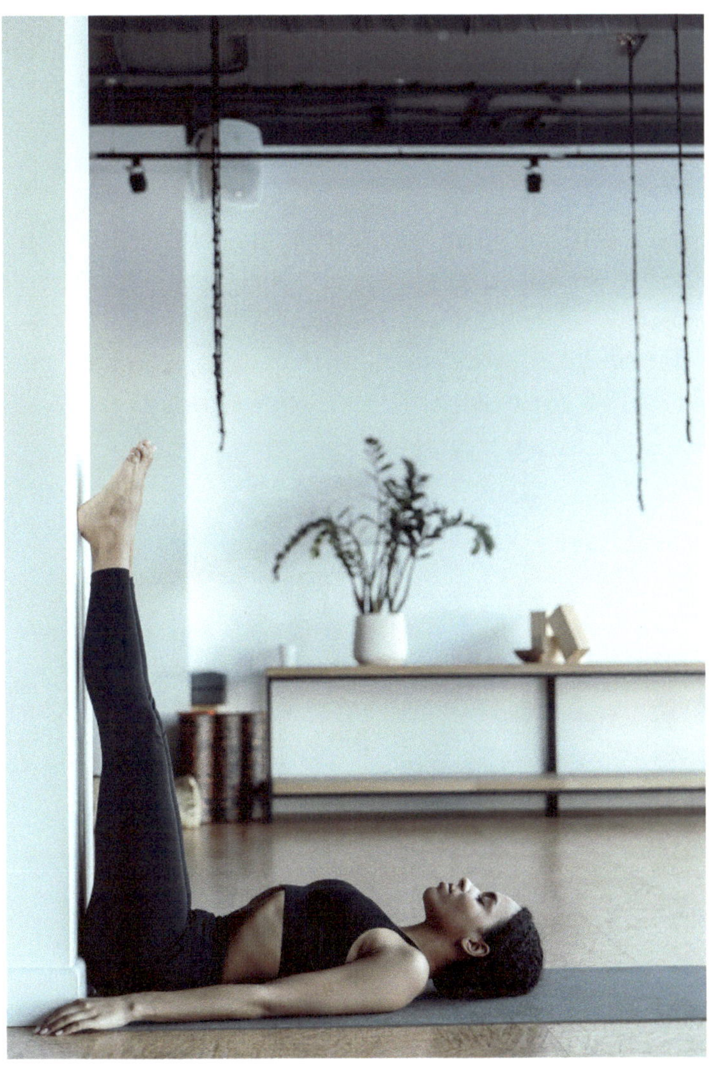

Child's Pose (Balasana)

The Child's Pose is a restful pose that allows you to turn inward and focus on your breath.

Instructions:

Start by kneeling on your mat, with your knees wider than your hips.
Sit back on your heels and fold forward, extending your arms in front of you.
Rest your forehead on the mat and breathe deeply.
Modifications: If your forehead doesn't reach the mat, you can stack your fists or use a block to support it.

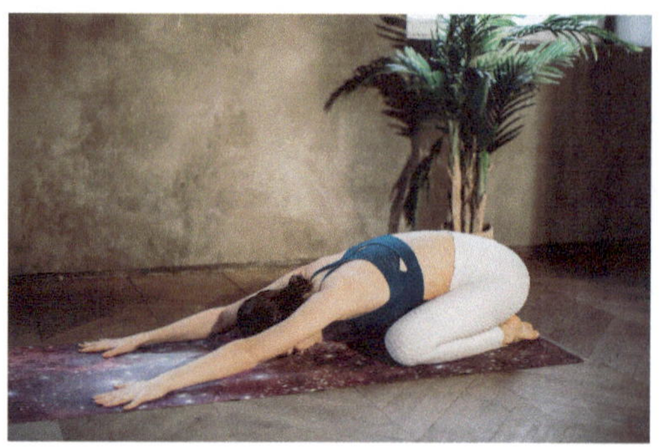

Corpse Pose (Savasana)

The Corpse Pose is typically the final pose in a yoga practice, allowing your body and mind to absorb the benefits of your practice.

Instructions:

Lie down on your back and let your legs and arms relax, with your palms facing up.
Close your eyes and take slow, deep breaths, allowing your body to relax and sink into the mat.
Modifications: If lying flat on your back is uncomfortable, you can place a rolled-up blanket or bolster under your knees.

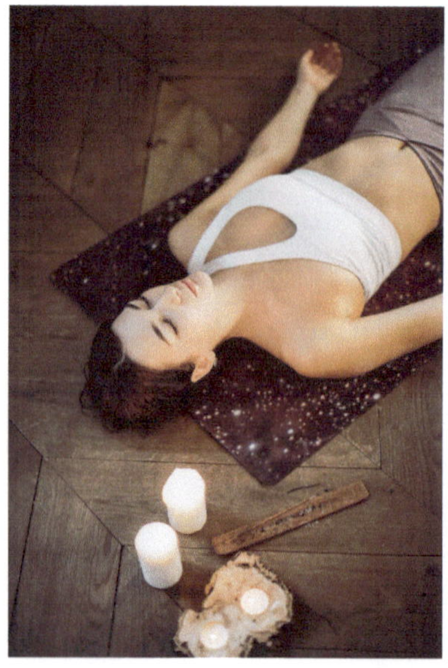

Remember, the goal of this sequence is relaxation and preparing for sleep. So, take your time, move slowly, and let your breath guide you. Sweet Dreams

Sequence Seven: Improving Posture

Introduction and Overview

Good posture isn't just about looking confident—it's crucial for your overall health and well-being. It helps keep your bones and joints in alignment, reduces the risk of back pain, and even improves your breathing. This sequence is designed to help you stand taller and feel better, with poses that strengthen your back and core and open up your chest.

Mountain Pose (Tadasana)
The Mountain Pose is a simple standing pose that helps you find alignment and balance.

Instructions:

Stand tall with your feet hip-width apart.
Press your feet into the ground and engage your leg muscles.
Lengthen your spine and roll your shoulders back and down.
Reach your fingertips towards the ground and lift the crown of your head towards the sky.
Modifications: If standing for a long time is uncomfortable, feel free to take breaks and shake out your legs.

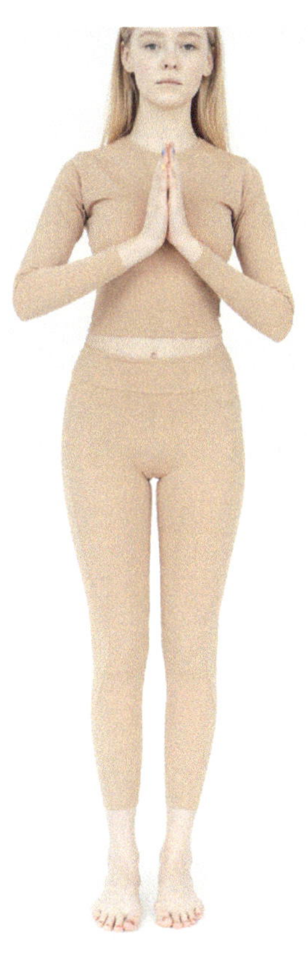

Cobra Pose (Bhujangasana)
The Cobra Pose is a gentle backbend that strengthens your back and opens up your chest.

Instructions:

Lie on your stomach with your hands under your shoulders.
Press your hands into the mat and lift your chest off the floor, keeping your hips and legs grounded.
Keep a slight bend in your elbows and open your chest forward.
Modifications: If this feels too intense, you can keep your forearms on the ground for a gentler backbend.

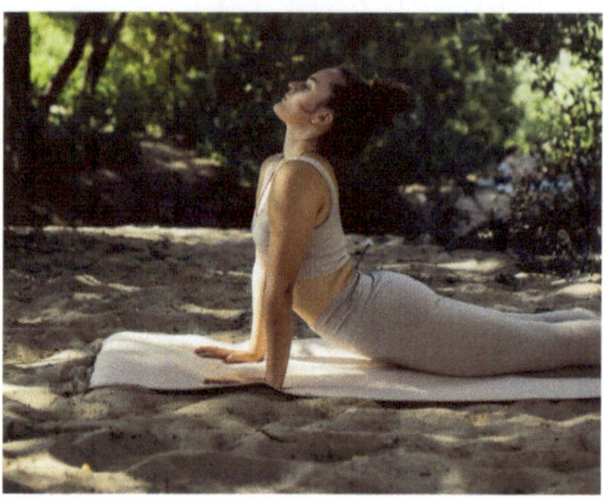

Bridge Pose (Setu Bandha Sarvangasana)
The Bridge Pose is a backbend that strengthens your back and opens up your chest and shoulders.

Instructions:

Lie on your back with your knees bent and your feet flat on the floor, hip-width apart.
Press your feet and arms into the floor and lift your hips towards the ceiling.
If it feels comfortable, you can clasp your hands under your body and roll your shoulders under to lift your hips higher.
Modifications: If lifting your hips is too much, you can keep them on the ground and focus on pressing your lower back into the floor.

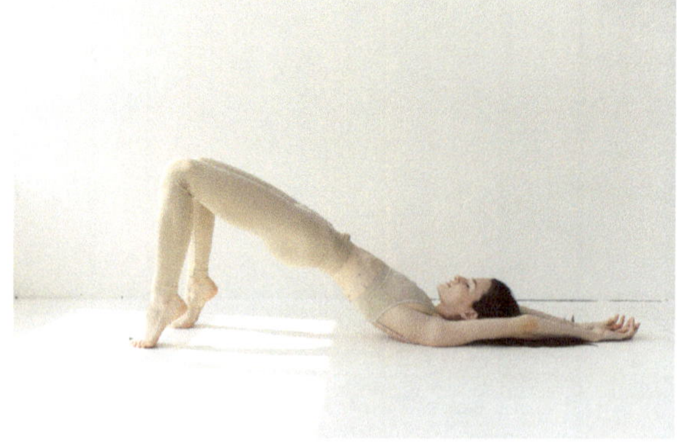

Remember, improving your posture is a gradual process, so be patient with yourself. Practice these poses regularly, and over time, you'll start to notice a difference in how you stand and move. Enjoy the journey!

Sequence Eight: Opening the Hips

Introduction and Overview

If you spend a lot of time sitting, whether at a desk job or during a long commute, your hips might feel tight or stiff. But don't worry—you're not alone, and yoga can help. This sequence is designed to gently open your hips, releasing tension and improving flexibility.

Butterfly Pose (Baddha Konasana)

The Butterfly Pose is a seated pose that opens your hips and stretches your inner thighs.

Instructions:

Sit on your mat with your knees bent and the soles of your feet together.
Hold onto your feet or ankles and sit up tall.
Gently press your knees down towards the floor, but don't force them.
Modifications: If your knees are high off the ground, you can sit on a cushion or block to elevate your hips.

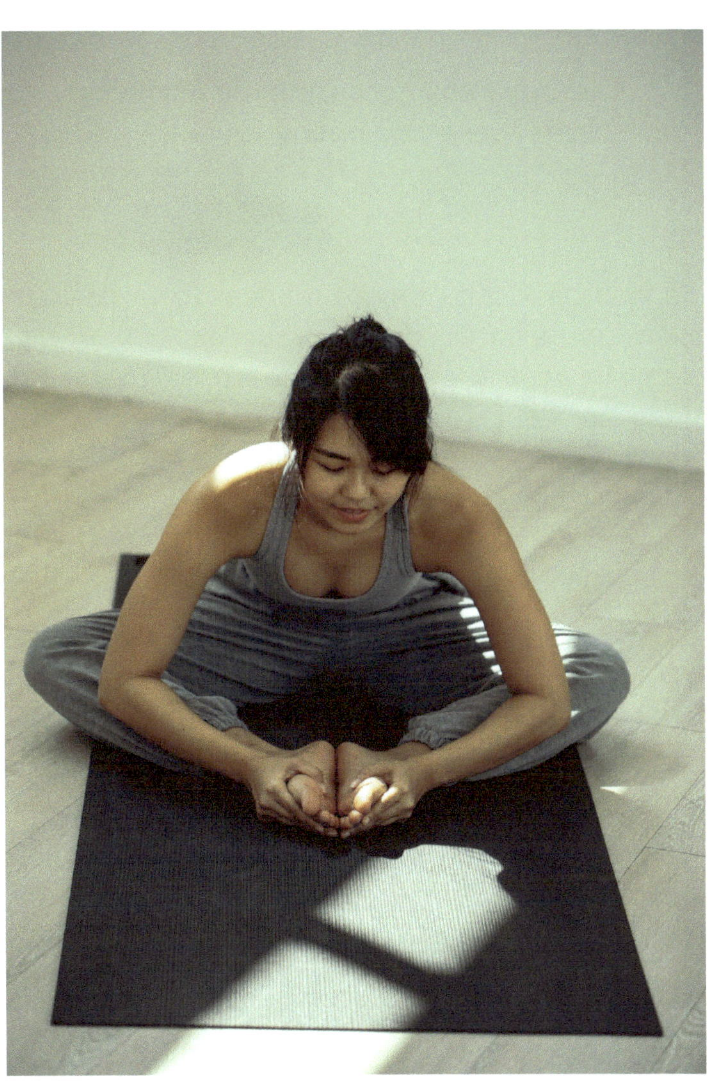

Pigeon Pose (Eka Pada Rajakapotasana)
The Pigeon Pose is a deep hip opener that also stretches your thighs and groin.

Instructions:

Start in a tabletop position, then bring your right knee forward towards your right wrist.
Extend your left leg behind you and square your hips to the front of your mat.
Stay upright or fold forward over your right leg, depending on what feels best for you.
Modifications: If this pose is too intense, you can place a block or folded blanket under your right hip for support.

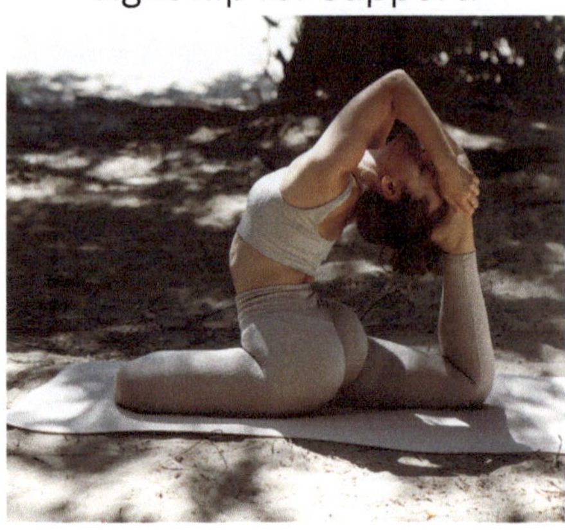

Happy Baby Pose (Ananda Balasana)
The Happy Baby Pose is a playful pose that opens your hips and gently stretches your back.

Instructions:

Lie on your back and bring your knees towards your chest.
Hold onto the outer edges of your feet or your big toes.
Gently pull your knees towards the floor beside your torso, keeping your back flat on the mat.
Modifications: If holding your feet is too much, you can hold onto your ankles or the backs of your thighs instead.

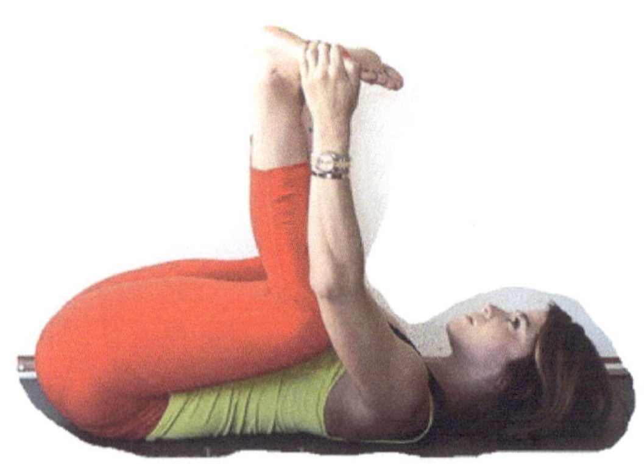

Remember, hip opening is a gradual process, so be patient with yourself. Practice these poses regularly, and over time, you'll start to notice a difference in your hip flexibility. Enjoy the journey!

Yoga for Better Sleep

Introduction

Sleep is essential for our health and well-being, but many of us struggle to get the quality rest we need. That's where yoga comes in. Yoga can help calm the mind, relax the body, and prepare you for a good night's sleep. The gentle stretching can relieve physical tension, while the focus on breath and mindfulness can help quiet the mind.

Sequence for Better Sleep

Child's Pose (Balasana)

Start on your hands and knees. Spread your knees wide apart while keeping your big toes touching. Rest your buttocks on your heels. Sit up straight and lengthen your spine up through the crown of your head.
On an exhalation, bow forward, draping your torso between your thighs. Your heart and chest should rest between or on top of your thighs. Allow your forehead to come to the floor.
Benefits: This pose helps to relax the body and calm the mind, preparing you for sleep.
Precautions: If you have a knee injury, avoid this pose unless you have the supervision of an experienced teacher.
Modifications: If it's difficult to sit on your heels in this pose, you can place a thickly folded blanket between your back thighs and calves.

Legs-Up-The-Wall Pose (Viparita Karani)

Sit next to a wall and swing your legs up onto the wall as you lay down on your back. Your body should form a 90-degree angle with the wall.
Extend your arms out to the sides and relax into the pose, keeping your legs as straight as possible.
Benefits: This pose can help to relax the body and mind, reduce anxiety, and prepare you for sleep.
Precautions: If you have serious eye problems, such as glaucoma, avoid this pose.
Modifications: If it's uncomfortable to have your legs straight up the wall, you can place a bend in your knees or move a little further away from the wall.

Corpse Pose (Savasana)

Lie flat on your back with your arms at your sides, palms facing up. Close your eyes and take slow, deep breaths.
Allow your body to feel heavy and sink into the floor, releasing all tension.
Benefits: This pose helps to relax the body, calm the mind, and reduce stress and anxiety, preparing you for sleep.
Precautions: If you're pregnant, lie on your left side instead of on your back.
Modifications: If it's uncomfortable to lie flat, you can place a rolled-up blanket under your knees to relieve any tension in the lower back.

Remember, yoga is not about striving for perfection—it's about connecting with yourself and finding peace and relaxation. So, take your time, listen to your body, and enjoy the journey towards better sleep.

Yoga for Stress Relief

Introduction

In our fast-paced world, stress is a common issue that can impact our health and well-being. Yoga, with its focus on mindful movement and deep breathing, can be an effective way to manage and reduce stress. The following sequence is designed to help you release tension, calm your mind, and find a sense of peace and relaxation.

Sequence for Stress Relief

Cat-Cow Pose (Marjaryasana-Bitilasana)

Start on your hands and knees in a tabletop position. Make sure your knees are set directly below your hips and your wrists, elbows, and shoulders are in line and perpendicular to the floor.
As you inhale, lift your sitting bones and chest toward the ceiling, allowing your belly to sink toward the floor (Cow Pose).
As you exhale, round your spine toward the ceiling, making sure to keep your shoulders and knees in position (Cat Pose).
Benefits: This pose helps to relieve tension in the spine and neck, promotes a sense of relaxation, and helps to massage the organs.
Precautions: If you have a neck injury, keep your head in line with your torso throughout the pose.
Modifications: If you have difficulty with this pose, you can modify it by placing a folded blanket under your knees.

Seated Forward Bend (Paschimottanasana)

Sit on the floor with your buttocks supported on a folded blanket and your legs straight in front of you. Press actively through your heels.
Inhale, and keeping the front torso long, lean forward from the hip joints. If possible, take the sides of the feet with your hands.
Stay in the pose anywhere from 1 to 3 minutes.
Benefits: This pose helps to calm the brain, relieve stress and mild depression, and stretch the spine, shoulders, and hamstrings.
Precautions: If you have asthma or diarrhea, avoid this pose. If you have a back injury, only perform this pose under the supervision of an experienced teacher.
Modifications: If you have a back injury, do this pose with bent knees, or perform it by lying on your back, with your thighs into your torso, your knees bent, and your feet on the floor.

Corpse Pose (Savasana)

Lie on your back with your legs straight and arms at your sides. Rest your hands about six inches away from your body with your palms up. Let your feet drop open. Close your eyes.
Let your breath occur naturally. Allow your body to feel heavy.
Stay in Savasana for five minutes for every 30 minutes of your practice.
Benefits: This pose helps to calm the brain, relieve stress, and relax the body.
Precautions: If you're pregnant, lie on your left side instead of on your back.
Modifications: If it's uncomfortable to lie flat, you can place a rolled-up blanket under your knees to relieve any tension in the lower back.

Remember, the goal of this sequence is to help you find a sense of peace and relaxation. Take your time, listen to your body, and let go of any judgment or expectations. You're doing great!

Yoga for Energy and Focus

Introduction

We all have those days when we feel sluggish or distracted. Instead of reaching for another cup of coffee, why not try yoga? Yoga can help to wake up your body, sharpen your mind, and boost your energy levels. The following sequence is designed to invigorate you and help you find your focus.

Sequence for Energy and Focus

Downward-Facing Dog (Adho Mukha Svanasana)

Start on your hands and knees. Align your wrists directly under your shoulders and your knees under your hips.
Press your hands into the floor and lift your hips back and up, straightening your legs as much as possible.
Keep your head between your arms and press your chest towards your thighs.
Benefits: This pose energizes the body, stretches the shoulders, hamstrings, and calves, and strengthens the arms and legs.
Precautions: If you have carpal tunnel syndrome, high blood pressure, a detached retina, or are in late-term pregnancy, modify this pose or avoid it.
Modifications: If it's hard to lift your hips, keep your knees on the floor and focus on lengthening your spine.

Warrior II Pose (Virabhadrasana II)

Stand with your feet wide apart. Turn your right foot out 90 degrees and your left foot in slightly.
Extend your arms out to the sides and bend your right knee, aligning it directly over your right ankle.
Gaze out over your right hand and breathe deeply.
Benefits: This pose strengthens the legs and arms, opens the chest and shoulders, and increases stamina.
Precautions: If you have high blood pressure, heart problems, or are suffering from diarrhea, avoid this pose.
Modifications: If it's hard to hold this pose, you can use a wall to support your back.

Tree Pose (Vrksasana)

Stand tall and balance on your right foot. Bring your left foot to rest against your right inner thigh or calf (but not your knee).
Bring your hands together in prayer position at your chest, or extend them above your head.
Focus on a point in front of you and breathe deeply.
Benefits: This pose strengthens the legs, improves balance, and promotes concentration and focus.
Precautions: If you have high blood pressure, practice this pose with your hands at your chest, not overhead.
Modifications: If it's hard to balance, you can stand with your back against a wall, or use a chair for support.

Remember, yoga is not about perfection—it's about connecting with yourself and finding what feels good. So, take your time, listen to your body, and enjoy the energy boost!

Yoga for Better Posture

Introduction

In our modern world, many of us spend hours each day sitting at a desk, staring at a computer screen, which can lead to slouching and poor posture. But don't worry, yoga can help. Yoga strengthens the core, lengthens the spine, and promotes better body awareness, which all contribute to improved posture. The following sequence is designed to help you stand taller and feel more confident.

Sequence for Better Posture

Mountain Pose (Tadasana)

Stand tall with your feet hip-width apart and your arms at your sides.
Press your weight evenly across all four corners of both feet.
Lengthen your spine and reach the crown of your head up towards the ceiling, while keeping your shoulders relaxed.
Benefits: This pose improves posture, strengthens the thighs, knees, and ankles, and reduces flat feet.
Precautions: If you have a headache, insomnia, low blood pressure, or if you are dizzy, practice this pose with the support of a wall.
Modifications: If standing is difficult, you can practice this pose sitting in a chair.

Cobra Pose (Bhujangasana)

Lie on your stomach with your hands under your shoulders and your fingers pointing forward.
Press your hands into the mat and slowly lift your chest off the floor, keeping your lower ribs on the mat.
Keep your elbows close to your body and your shoulders away from your ears.
Benefits: This pose strengthens the spine, stretches the chest and lungs, and helps to improve posture.
Precautions: Avoid this pose if you have a back injury, carpal tunnel syndrome, or are pregnant.
Modifications: If it's hard to lift your chest, you can keep your elbows on the floor and gently lift your chest as far as is comfortable.

Bridge Pose (Setu Bandha Sarvangasana)

Lie on your back with your knees bent and your feet flat on the floor, hip-width apart.
Press your feet and arms into the floor and lift your hips towards the ceiling.
Keep your thighs parallel and your knees directly over your ankles.
Benefits: This pose strengthens the back, buttocks, and hamstrings, improves circulation, and helps to improve posture.
Precautions: Avoid this pose if you have a neck injury.
Modifications: If it's hard to lift your hips, you can place a block or bolster under your sacrum for support.

Remember, improving your posture is a gradual process, so be patient with yourself. Practice these poses regularly, and over time, you'll start to notice a difference in your posture and alignment. Stand tall and be proud!

Creating a Consistent Practice

The Importance of Consistency

Consistency is key in any form of exercise, and yoga is no exception. Regular practice can help you reap the full benefits of yoga, from increased flexibility and strength to improved mental clarity and stress reduction. In fact, research has shown that consistent yoga practice can lead to significant improvements in health and well-being. So, while it might be tempting to only roll out your mat when you're in the mood, try to make yoga a regular part of your routine.

Creating a Routine

Creating a routine might sound daunting, but it doesn't have to be. Start by finding a regular time for your yoga practice. It could be first thing in the morning to set a positive tone for the day, during your lunch break to recharge, or in the evening to wind down before bed. Next, create a dedicated yoga space. It doesn't have to be a large or fancy space - just a quiet spot where you won't be disturbed. Having a dedicated space can help signal to your brain that it's time for yoga.

Finding Motivation

Staying motivated can be a challenge, especially when you're just starting out. One way to stay motivated is by setting achievable goals. Maybe you want to be able to touch your toes, hold a plank for a minute, or simply feel more relaxed and focused. Tracking your progress can also be a powerful motivator. Consider keeping a yoga journal to note how you feel after each practice, any progress you've made, and any insights or inspirations that come up during your practice.

Overcoming Barriers

One of the most common barriers to a consistent yoga practice is a lack of time. But remember, even a short practice is better than no practice. If you're pressed for time, try doing a quick 5-minute sequence or even a single pose. You'd be surprised how much difference it can make. Lack of space can also be a barrier, but remember, all you really need is enough space to lay out a yoga mat. You can do yoga in your living room, your bedroom, or even outdoors.

Remember, the goal is not to create a perfect practice, but a consistent one. Be patient with yourself, listen to your body, and most importantly, enjoy the journey. Happy practicing!

Conclusion

As we come to the end of this guide, let's take a moment to reflect on what we've covered. We've explored the origins and principles of yoga, and how it can fit into our busy modern lives. We've learned about the physical and mental benefits of yoga, from improved flexibility and strength to reduced stress and better sleep. We've gone through eight short yoga sequences, each designed to be completed in just five minutes, and targeted sequences for specific needs like better sleep, stress relief, energy and focus, and improved posture. And finally, we've discussed the importance of consistency in yoga practice and shared practical tips for creating a routine, finding motivation, and overcoming common barriers.

But remember, this is just the beginning of your yoga journey. The true magic of yoga lies in its long-term benefits, which can only be experienced through consistent practice. So, I encourage you to keep going. Roll out your mat, even if it's just for five minutes a day. Listen to your body, honor your progress, and most importantly, enjoy the process. Yoga is not about perfection—it's about connection, with your body, your mind, and your spirit.

I would love to hear about your experiences with this guide. Did you find the sequences helpful? Have you noticed any changes in your body or mind since you started practicing regularly? Your feedback is invaluable and can help improve future editions of this book.

Thank you for joining me on this yoga journey. Remember, every time you step onto your mat, you're taking a step towards better health and well-being. Keep going, and enjoy the journey. Namaste.

References/Resources

As we wrap up this guide, I'd like to leave you with some additional resources to help you continue your yoga journey. These are some of my favorite yoga channels, apps, books, and online courses that have inspired and supported me in my own practice:

Yoga Channels:

"Yoga with Adriene": Adriene Mishler's approachable and down-to-earth yoga videos are perfect for beginners.
"Fightmaster Yoga": Lesley Fightmaster offers a wide range of yoga classes, from gentle Hatha to more challenging Ashtanga sequences.

Yoga Apps:

"Down Dog": This app offers customizable yoga practices, making it easy to fit yoga into your day, no matter how much time you have.
"Insight Timer": In addition to guided meditations, this app offers a variety of yoga classes and courses.

Books:

"Light on Yoga" by B.K.S. Iyengar: This classic book provides detailed instructions and illustrations for a wide range of yoga poses.
"The Yoga Bible" by Christina Brown: A comprehensive guide to yoga practice with over 150 yoga poses.
Online Courses:

"Yoga Fundamentals" on Coursera: This course offers a deep dive into the principles and practice of yoga.
"Yoga for Well-being" on Udemy: This course focuses on using yoga for stress relief, improved flexibility, and overall wellness.
Acknowledgments

I'd like to extend my deepest gratitude to everyone who has supported me in the creation of this book. Your encouragement and feedback have been invaluable.

If you have any questions or would like to share your experiences with this guide, please feel free to reach out to me at [author's email]. I look forward to hearing from you.

Remember, the journey of yoga is a personal one. Take what serves you, leave what doesn't, and always listen to your body. Happy practicing!